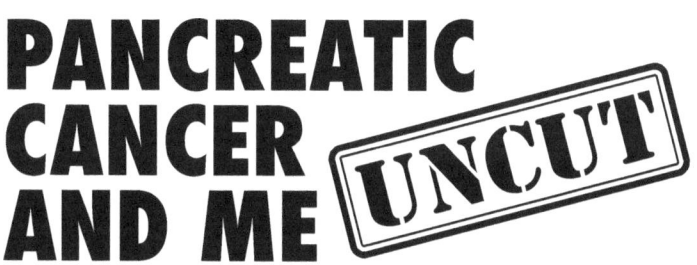

PANCREATIC CANCER AND ME UNCUT

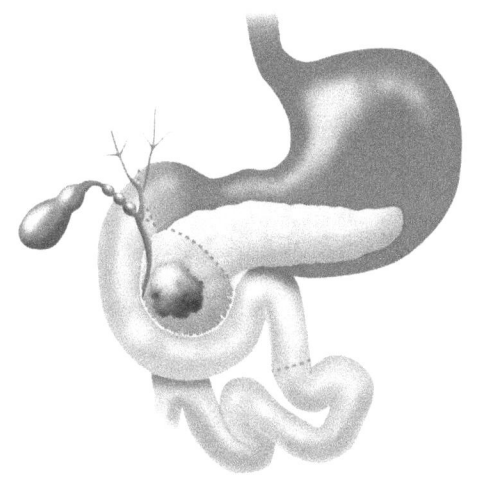

SAMSON BYRD

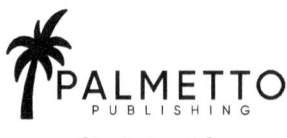

Charleston, SC
www.PalmettoPublishing.com

Pancreatic Cancer and Me, Uncut

Copyright © 2022

by Samson Byrd

All rights reserved

No portion of this book may be reproduced, stored in a retrieval system, or transmitted in any form by any means–electronic, mechanical, photocopy, recording, or other–except for brief quotations in printed reviews, without prior permission of the author.

First Edition

Paperback ISBN: 979-8-88590-161-1

CONTENTS

Foreword	1
Prediagnosis	3
The Hospital	13
The Diagnosis	19
My Treatment Plan	24
The Wonderment	62
Acknowledgment	67

FOREWORD

In *Pancreatic Cancer and Me, Uncut,* the author recalls his months of testing, trials, and tribulations he went through dealing with the battle of his life, the fight with pancreatic cancer. He holds nothing back. Uncut, he shares with grace and in detail his experiences from the onset of the disease to its diagnosis, progression, treatment, recovery, and finally, to trying to get his life back. Even while in pain, he tries to show compassion and a sense of humor and let you know it's okay to cry and call out to God for help and strength.

PREDIAGNOSIS

Routinely I was going about my daily living, attending church, doing the lawn, doing a little fishing now and then. I would travel a little. I would travel to New Orleans, Southern Mississippi along Interstate 55, and St. Louis, Missouri, and Southern Illinois to have fun with family and friends. I was alive! I was a "the party is over here" kind of guy even at seventy-one or seventy-two years of age. I felt strong, even though I had had two back surgeries, one traditional with the knife and the other one with laser.

Healthwise, I felt that my health was fair to okay. However, in 2016 I began to experience wheezing, sinus flare-ups, dark red eyes that would clear up and come again, and low oxygen levels. Some doctors said I had chronic obstructive pulmonary disease (COPD)—adult-onset asthma. I didn't like that call, so I told the doctor that I didn't smoke, nor did I ever have trouble with asthma. I was told that I didn't have to have smoked. The doctor then said to me that he didn't smoke either and that he suffered the same things.

I felt that all was wrong with me was that I had a bad sinus infection. So I went to an ear nose and throat (ENT) clinic. I told the doctor that I had been wheezing and had experienced low oxygen and dark red eyes. I let the doctor know that I was planning to get married in a few weeks. I was diagnosed with a bad sinus infection—sinusitis. I was prescribed some antibiotics and an inhaler for the wheezing. He looked at me and laughed. He said, "I want you to have plenty of air since you are getting married." I didn't get the meaning of that until I got home.

In a few days, I felt so much better. When I heard myself wheeze, I would puff the inhaler to solve that problem. I wanted to say to myself, I told the doctor that I didn't have COPD nor asthma, but I also told myself to be quiet on that issue.

In April 2016 I got married. I felt pretty well. I had a great wedding celebration with family and friends. I later reviewed several close-up photos of myself. I'm my best critic. I saw some photos that I didn't like that much because I appeared to be tired, red-eyed, dazed, and more overweight than I realized.

I went back to visit my wife's family and friends for the Christmas gathering. My brother-in-law had made a slide presentation that featured some of the photos of me from the wedding, where he told me that I looked a bit out of whack. I agreed and wished I could have erased one of the slides where I didn't look so well. My wife even commented that she felt perhaps I was having marriage remorse because of the way I was looking at times. Again I had to explain to her that I had been sick with low oxygen, sinusitis, and wheezing just a few weeks before our wedding. I had to rush to try to get better so I wouldn't have to use sickness as an excuse to change a planned and already-set date for our wedding.

It was perhaps Father's Day in June 2018 when I received a letter from my son in which he told me that he was going to make me proud of him one day. That sounded somewhat strange and awkward to me. I hadn't heard anything like that coming from him before. So I wondered deeply to try to understand what he was really saying to me. Did he think that I somehow felt that he had let me down or disappointed me? The days of my suggesting to him things he could do, what college or university to attend, or what field of study to pursue were long gone. I still wondered what he really meant, and I tried hard to figure it out.

I told a clergy friend what my son said to me, thinking he could help me interpret it. His reply was, "Just tell your son that you love him and that you have always been proud of him." The daddy in me wouldn't let me do that. I figured he should have known that by now. I did ask him periodically how he was doing. He would tell me he was doing fine and still in school. At that time that was very satisfactory to me and made me very proud of him with no further questions asked.

Then, in early 2019 another letter came from him telling that he had graduation dates for me—May 15 and 17, 2019. Wow, immediately I started to plan to be there. Was this what he meant when he said one day he would make me proud of him?

By mid-2018 I began to notice that my back bothered me more, and I began to detect weakness in my left leg. I used my walking cane more to perhaps prevent a stumble or fall. When I was asked, "What are you doing with that cane?" I would smile and reply, "My cane needs me more than I need it." This early-seventy-year-old man was beginning to notice changes in his health that were becoming more noticeable and more frequent. Residual problems associated with my service-connected back problems, such as neuropathy, numbness and tingling in both feet, tiredness, and pressure pushing downward across the center of my back were getting me down.

I sought medical help for these problems. I would be prescribed gabapentin, ibuprofen, tramadol, and Toradol shots. I was told that I was a candidate for back surgery, where a rod would be placed in my back. Such an operation would have left me with severe pain and stiffness for a whole year. It was up to me to opt in or opt out.

My back episode got worse. I was sent to an imaging clinic for an MRI of the back. My back was so inflamed I couldn't lie on that cold, flat surface to finish the MRI scan. I returned to my primary doctor for further care. I was also seeing a urologist. I had been told that my testosterone was low. I was getting testosterone shots monthly. Each time I checked in for the shots, it seemed that my blood pressure would be slightly elevated. Mind you, I had been told of a graduation date in May 2019.

The intensity and frequency of my health issues became more apparent. It seemed that my weight was sneaking up on me. I felt like everything I ate went directly to my belly fat. At times I would get fatigued. I would catch myself falling asleep while waiting for the signal light to change. The most bizarre thing that even made me laugh at myself was when I caught myself a couple of times sleeping on my zero-turn mower just going around in circles like a Jet Ski in my yard. What was that all about? I don't know. I only hoped that my wife hadn't peeked out a window and seen me doing that. I felt bloat-y and full of gas, especially after I ate. I told myself many times that I probably needed to go to a gastroenterologist. I never did it. I would rationalize by saying to myself that I just had a colonoscopy, and the next one was not due until three years later.

It was now early 2019. I kept reminding myself I had to be well enough to attend my son's graduation. I became very gassy. I couldn't control it at night. I was a fairly newlywed. "Excuse me" is okay but not good enough when you are trying to get to know your new wife. I told my wife once when one partner can fart and both laugh about it, you have bonded and know each other. I could not control it. I would jump up out of bed to rush to the bathroom, farting each step of the way. When I got there, I would have enough gas to make a short tune by flexing my buttocks. Honey, I'm sorry, I can't help it. The farts just come by themselves. I do not try to do that. I don't know why.

I noticed that my urine had begun to turn dark and ugly looking. For some time I didn't say anything to my wife. I kept that to myself.

I figured it would clear up if I drank more water. Later I noticed that my urine seemed darker and heavier. It appeared as if the darker and heavier part of my urine would sink to the bottom of the toilet, while the lighter color would float over the heavier, darker color. Then I would say to my wife, "Honey, my urine looks dark and heavy." I tried to describe it as looking like a slightly used or burned motor oil. I was getting concerned about it. It just didn't look normal. I then told myself to tell the urologist about it since I was getting testosterone shots from him. He agreed to do a urine test.

The results came back showing everything was okay. I didn't feel good with those results. I went back to my primary care doctor to complain further about my health issues. I also explained that my back was so inflamed that I couldn't complete my MRI. Another issue I discussed was that my eyes would turn a dirty red color and last for some time. I would also get weird feelings like an anxiety attack. I felt like I had better go to the hospital to have myself checked for diabetes. I would ask my wife if she had some candy. At times I would say that I was not feeling well. The consensus would be "Let's go to the hospital."

I didn't want them to find anything or tell me that I was a diabetic. Yet I would be somewhat disappointed when tests would show normal blood pressure, sugar level, and oxygen level. I would be asked if my eyes were always that funny red color. A short time in the emergency room, I would be feeling fine and normal again. My comment would be "I am the healthiest sick man I know."

Later my primary care doctor called me in for a checkup. While there I informed the doctor that I couldn't complete the MRI exam of my back because of the pain of lying on the flat and cold table. I did the routine blood work, and I was X-rayed in a standing position with my back against the x-ray machine, and a side view of my back was made.

In March 2019 the breaking news was that Alex Trebek had been diagnosed with stage four pancreatic cancer. I had heard of such cancer, but it hadn't hit home with me. However, a man I grew up with and attended elementary and high school with, one I called my play brother, told me that the doctors told him that he had pancreatic cancer. I visited him in the hospital for diabetes and heart conditions. He was concerned why the doctors had just discovered he had pancreatic cancer when he had been going to them for a long period fighting diabetes and heart disease. I saw another young lady fighting the battle with cancer to later find out that she also had pancreatic cancer. I saw two others fight breast cancer. I felt empathy for those who were going through their pain. When I knew of those suffering with their sickness, I surely would visit them in the hospitals and their homes.

Now late April 2019 was approaching. I was making plans to attend my son's graduation in May 2019 in Fayetteville, North Carolina, some eight-hundred-plus miles away. Should I drive, or should I fly? I was wrestling with the idea. If I flew out there, that would create a getting-around problem. So I decided to drive. That way I would have my own transportation and could go and come as I pleased.

One midafternoon I received a call from my primary care doctor's office with some strange questions that caught me off guard. The person on the phone asked questions to verify who I was. After I was identified, she told me that my doctor had her to call me to ask if I was taking any over-the-counter drugs in addition to my prescribed medicines. I said no. There were a few other questions asked. My answer to all the questions was no. She said okay, and our conversation ended. I was now wondering what that was all about. Later the doctor herself called and asked to speak with me. She said, "I checked over your test results and saw that your liver enzymes are very high, even higher than at the first test results. Go now, straight to the emergency room!"

I was really curious now. I told my wife that the call was from my primary care doctor. My wife was anxious to know why. I said all I knew was that she said my liver enzymes were very high and that I had to go straight to the emergency room. Thinking and moving slowly, I headed for the shower and commenced putting on clean clothes and underwear. You know, my mother always taught me that when you go somewhere, have on clean underwear because you might have to go the hospital. Liver enzymes—I had never heard of such in all my years of living. I was not panicking, though, wondering what in the world I was getting ready to face as I drove to the hospital.

THE HOSPITAL

Earlier I had been at this hospital, and I saw a very crowded waiting room with people waiting to be seen. I saw people leaving because the wait had been so long. That was what I was anticipating, a long hurry-up-and-wait line. However, this time I had a great and timely experience. When I arrived at the hospital, I was immediately called in to be waited on, and quickly I was dressed in my hospital gown and whisked down the halls on a hospital gurney into x-ray and other imaging rooms for tests. I noticed all imaging was done on my abdominal area. When all the lab work and imaging were completed, I was sent home to report to my primary care doctor. She reviewed the scans and findings. I was then set up with an appointment to see a gastrointestinal doctor. From all the bloating and gas I had been experiencing, I told myself, "I told you that you needed to have your upper and lower stomach checked out." These are the kinds of things we tell ourselves to do, but we have a tendency to put them off.

The gastrointestinal doctor took a look at my imaging scans and findings. I was told, as I understood it, that I had a blockage that was effecting my liver and gallbladder, and there was a tumor at the head of my pancreas. All this happening was causing my urine to be very dark. At this time it was too early to say whether the tumor was cancerous. The doctor told me that he was going to put a stent in my stomach to relieve some of the blockage. At the same time, a biopsy would be done on the tumor to see whether it was cancerous.

The stent was placed in my stomach. I was told that it would take several days to get the pathology report back on the tumor biopsy. This occurred right about the time of my son's graduation. I conferred with my wife. I felt that this would allow me time to go and attend my son's graduation while waiting for the biopsy report. Therefore, I asked my gastrointestinal doctor if I could drive. Loosely, without eye contact, he said yes. I was well aware that my stomach was not acting right, with bloating, gas, and constipation. Also my urine was still dark and heavy looking. My eyes had begun to change to a noticeable green-yellowish look. Otherwise I felt okay. Though I wondered if I would be able to drive eight hundred miles one way to attend my son's graduation. Not knowing what the outcome of the biopsy would be, again, I asked the doctor if I could drive. Again, he said yes. I didn't tell him how far. *Yes* was what I wanted to hear. I didn't want to disappoint anyone.

My wife and I loaded up into my car. I was on my way to Fayetteville, North Carolina! While on the way, I began to itch and scratch my shoulders. I got frustrated. This itching episode was new. I was afraid to let my wife drive. I was scared of how she would do in rush hour and multilane traffic. Then when I was driving, it was, "Turn your signals off/on." "Don't get so close to the edge of the road." By the grace of God and his protection, we made it safely to Fayetteville.

On May 15, 2019, my son graduated from college as a registered nurse. I am grateful to God for allowing me to witness that event and allowing my son to witness my presence there. To my surprise, my son is now a registered nurse. His sister and mother are nurses also. My demeanor and countenance were being monitored by medical professionals as I was trying to put on my best face to act as if I was feeling my best when I really was feeling bad.

The postgraduation activities were great. I was now trying to get some rest in preparation for the long drive back to Mississippi. My son pulled me aside and told me that my daughter wanted to see me before I left for home. I wondered what that was all about. I made it over to her home, where the kids were playing and the barbecue grill was all fired up in the backyard. I tried to play with the kids and watched meat being turned on the grill. I wanted some of that food to boost my strength and provide me with a to-go plate.

I found the right moment to get my daughter alone to say, "I heard you wanted to talk to me. What's up?"

She looked at me and asked, "Are you all right? You don't look good! Is there something wrong?"

All I could do was drop my head. By this time all the adults' eyes and ears were focused on me, ready to see and hear what I had to say. I then told them just before my trip there, I had a CAT scan and MRI done on me. A stent had been placed in my stomach because there seemed to be a blockage that was not allowing the correct functioning of my gallbladder, kidneys, and liver. This had been the root cause of my dark urine and yellowing eyes. Also there had been a tumor found on or around the head my pancreas. They had done a biopsy of it, and I wouldn't know the results until I got back home. Now the cat was out of the bag. My family began to see and feel my pain. I was told perhaps I should not have made that long drive. My son said, "If you were sick, I would have understood if you hadn't come to my graduation." In my heart I was obligated to attend the graduation.

With my to-go plate in hand, I went back to my hotel to try to rest for the eight-hundred-mile trip home. We left early, before daybreak. I wanted to time and pace myself to arrive home early evening before dark. I was itching, scratching, and feeling constipated. My wife was also tired and frustrated with little or no rest from seeing me go through the agony. At daybreak I stopped at the first Walmart parking lot I could find. My wife wanted to know why we were stopping. I said I just needed to stop and lay my head against the window and try to sleep for a few minutes. My wife was telling me that she could drive. I was afraid of that. I was in such agony that I wanted to leave my car parked at Walmart and get a flight to Memphis. It was a crazy idea, but the agony of itching, scratching, and constipation put such a thought on my mind. I even wondered if what I was going through was some of the same affliction that Satan put on Job.

I managed to have a difficult bowel movement while at Walmart. I purchased a few bottles of those colored waters that had Pedialyte in them to hydrate me. Those and the bowel movement made me feel a bit better. Now I was well on my way home.

I got on a stretch of an interstate that was beautiful, in wide-open country among Alabama, Mississippi, and Tennessee. My wife said again that she was wide awake and could drive some. I was feeling somewhat better. Since we had bright sunshine and a clear, wide, and uncluttered interstate to drive on, I agreed to let her drive so that I could try to relax a bit. Like I planned it, we arrived home before dark. I thanked God for a safe trip to and fro. I also thanked God for giving me the strength to endure the agony and pain of the trip. Most of all I was grateful to God for allowing me to experience seeing my son graduate as a registered nurse.

THE DIAGNOSIS

My focus now was on the results of the biopsy and to find out why I was having so much problem with my bowels, itching, scratching, having constipation, experiencing yellowing of the eyes, and having dark urine. I returned to the gastrointestinal doctor for answers. I was told the tumor was found to be malignant. That stunned me to the point that I had to contrast benign with malignant to make sure I had the right meaning. In other words the tumor was found to be cancerous. It was located around the head of the pancreas, near some critical blood vessels. It was explained to me this was causing my eyes to yellow and my urine to be dark. I was still stunned but not alarmed or afraid. Nothing like this had ever happened to me before. I was told that I had pancreatic cancer. I asked the symptoms of such cancer. I was told none. It was pointed out to me that anytime one passes sixty years of age, one could look for something like this or anything else to happen to them. My diagnosis came in May 2019, just two months after Alex Trebek's diagnosis. I was told that I would have to see a surgeon.

I went home itching and scratching. I felt like little demons were trying to tear out from inside and puncture through my skin. I felt bumps and pimples popping out on my skin, especially on my arms, shoulders, and back. Constipation was harsh, and my stool became ugly. Sometimes it would look like coffee grounds. I went for further testing. My skin had become very tough like cowhide. Instead of a stick, several nurses who did blood work had to stab me with the needle. They would try and retry to draw blood. At times they would call for help to get a needle into my arm, which required a second and third painful stab. When a needle was finally inserted, then my vein would roll, requiring the painful process again.

Initially the process to see a surgeon seemed a bit slow. The first doctor showed me a beautiful colored eight-by-ten photo of a full internal stomach, showing the liver, gallbladder, large and small in-

THE DIAGNOSIS

testines, and pancreas. He appeared to be unsure whether he would be my doctor. In the photo he showed what would be done to me in a surgical situation for this cancer. I didn't see him again. A little frustrated, my wife made a few phone calls. I was given an appointment with another surgeon. When I met with him, the first thing he said was, "I hear you have been getting the run-around." He also stated that that would not happen again. He assured me that he would take care of me. He did just what he said.

Things got to moving with a sense of urgency. The first thing he did was put me on a table. He put one hand to my stomach and tapped it with the other hand. Immediately he said to me the stent that had been placed in my stomach was not working. How he knew that from just a tap is still a mystery to me. Quickly I was set up to have the original plastic stent removed and replaced with a heavier metal type. Things were moving faster now. As soon as it was done, I had another appointment with the surgeon. It was confirmed to me again that I had pancreatic cancer. He assured me again that he was going to take care of me. He told me that he was putting a team together to treat me. I told him, "Doc, I've already prayed for your team." When he told me that the original stent was not working only by tapping on my stomach, it was my confirmation that I had the right surgeon. He then told me the next step would be with the oncologist. He said that I was going to like her. Oncologist—wow, what a word. I had seen the word someplace, but I didn't know what an oncologist did. Before seeing the oncologist, I got a new stent placed in my stomach. This was an outpatient procedure.

As all this was taking place, the diagnosis of pancreatic cancer was beginning to sink in. My weight loss became more apparent to me. I noticed that I could pull my forty-six-inch-waist pants up over other clothing with them zipped and buttoned up. I was still itching, scratching, and suffering constipation. I didn't look well at all when I looked in the mirror. My nights were restless and miserable. My illness was getting into my head. I wanted to think negatively. But whenever I did, I would remember that my primary doctor told me to always think positively. She told me staying positive would be a huge part of my fight. I took that advice the best that I could.

I had more and more blood work done on me as well as another MRI and CAT scan. A port was placed in my chest. I had no idea what that was or what that meant until later. When I saw the port, I remembered that I had seen one of those things hanging out of my cousin's chest. He wanted to know where he could go and have it flushed. I had no idea what in the world he was talking about. Oh boy! I do now. Later, through inquiry, I found out my first cousin had cancer. I didn't even know it.

MY TREATMENT PLAN

My surgeon told me that his plan of treatment would last approximately one year. That took a big swallow for me to digest. Wow, for a whole year I would be going through the shadows of death. All I could do was be positive and pray. Now I had my appointment to meet with my oncologist. On the day of my appointment, I anxiously sat in the oncologist's office, waiting to be seen. I remembered the surgeon told me that I would like her. After a few minutes' wait, I heard a knock on the door. In stepped this tall, slender, dark lady. She pleasantly greeted me and announced that she was going to be my oncologist and she would be directing my chemotherapy proce-

MY TREATMENT PLAN

dures. I was examined, and then she reviewed my blood work. She counseled me in several areas. I was given a feel of what to expect. All I heard was totally strange and new to me. I didn't have sense enough to be afraid. I was comforted and told again not to worry and to be positive that I would get through this. My layman's evaluation of what I was hearing gave me full confidence in this beautiful, tall, dark oncologist. As the surgeon had told me, I did like her and said secretly to myself, "She sounds like she knows her stuff." I also said to myself, "Somebody has been lying to us. Black folks don't get into this kind of profession."

The analogy of my treatment would be like that of building a sandwich. The first slice of bread would be this office visit and various briefings, followed by several treatments of chemo by infusion, blood work, CAT scans, and evaluations. After several treatments of chemotherapy, I would then have several weeks of daily radiation therapy, coupled with chemo pills and evaluation. The meat of the sandwich would be a visit back to the surgeon for evaluation. The top slice would include a decision that I had to make, followed by a last round of chemotherapy. Now I must work this very difficult plan. I had been diagnosed with pancreatic cancer, a deadly and aggressive demonic cancer. I was still itching, and my eyes were still yellowish.

My bowels were still acting up, and my urine was still dark. I was a sick man with a lot of unknowns. This was the start of my chemotherapy treatments.

PHASE ONE: CHEMOTHERAPY

I WAS WHISKED INTO AN INFUSION room, where I had to verify the date of my birth and my name on bags of chemo medication. I was asked if I had a port. The answer was yes. For the first time, I understood what this thing, a port implanted in my chest, was to be used for. Boy, it saved me from sticks into my skin, which had become very tough. I would hear, "On three take a deep breath," and immediately I would be infusion-ready. An infusion session would take four to four-and-a-half hours, then I would be fitted with an infusion pump to be worn from Tuesday evening until Thursday around midday, at which time I would be cut loose from that apparatus for a few days. I would test my physical strength. I would be weak in my legs. My weight was falling rapidly. I couldn't touch or drink anything cold. The chemo was kicking my behind. My stomach was in turmoil. I got nauseated but couldn't throw up. I was constipated.

MY TREATMENT PLAN

I was so compacted that I would sweat trying to have a bowel movement. No joke, I prayed, "Lord, you said you would be an ever-present help in times of trouble." There were times I had to pray for help and strength to have a bowel movement.

It was now time to return for my second infusion. The first thing after check-in would be the "On three take a deep breath," followed by blood work and being made infusion-ready. I would have a CAT scan with contrast to see what was happening to me internally. After a brief wait for results, I again would be seen and evaluated by my oncologist. She wanted to know how I was feeling after my first chemotherapy treatment. It was the same story—constipation, itching, nausea, yellowing of the eyes, and dark urine.

"Doc, can you please give me something to quench this itching and constipation?" was my plea. "Doc, I also need something to help me sleep."

She would evaluate my blood work and go over some of the things with me, such as my blood cells, red to white, glucose level, kidney function, and so on, to name a few things.

The next question I had was, "Doc, why am I still itching so?" I explained that I couldn't sleep because of it. I had to sit up in a recliner because I disturbed my wife at night. (Our caregivers—in my case, my wife—are a gift from God.)

She told me that my bilirubin level was high.

I said, "Billy who? Can you please spell that for me?"

She said, "Bilirubin. It's high, but it is lower now than when you first came in. Otherwise, things are looking okay, and your numbers are moving in the right directions." She explained to me that she took it somewhat easy on me with the first infusion, but this time, in so many words, she stated that she was not going to be so lenient. I got the full blast of chemo the second time around.

The process repeated itself for a few weeks. Somewhere around my third or fourth treatment, I began to look at and notice myself in the mirror to observe how I was looking and feeling. I talked first to myself, then to my wife so she could verify what I was feeling and seeing of myself. I would let my wife know that the itching and scratching had begun to let up just a little bit. I also let her know that I was resting a bit better at night. She acknowledged that she had noticed I was resting better too. The mirror showed me that my eyes were looking better. The yellowish-greenish color was giving way to a more normal eye color. I was drinking more water, my urine was becoming lighter in color, and my skin tone was looking better. The other side of this, I noticed, was my weight was dropping rapidly. Over a short period, I went down from 270 pounds to around 216 pounds. My tongue and gums became dark and black. My fingernails turned dark, and the palms of my hands became black like the sole of a raccoon's foot.

In addition to talking to myself and my wife, I talked to God. I had to surrender and let him know here I was, diagnosed with what was called pancreatic cancer. I told him that I needed his strength to get me through this ordeal, a trial that I didn't know anything about. The only times I had been hospitalized were for a broken leg and back surgery. I can truly say that I am so glad that I had believed in and accepted Christ as my Lord and Savior before my diagnosis and treatments. I was active with my relationship with him. Therefore, I could pray for his strength to get me through my trials and not so much to get me out of them.

During my chemotherapy and infusion treatments, I, at times, had enough strength to go to my place of worship, where I assembled together with other members. My pastor was very active and was highly sought after to preach here and there. At times he would ask his members to go with him for support. That was my pastor. Naturally, when I had the strength and felt good enough to go, I would go. He would point me out to the congregation where he was preaching to let them know that I was one of his members. He informed them that I had been diagnosed with pancreatic cancer and was going through treatments for the deadly disease. Wow! That became another instant cloud of witnesses praying for me, encouraging me, and strengthening me.

I heard others tell me their testimonials of how their loved ones suffered the same or similar diseases. I was given examples of how they coped and dealt with their pain. One guy told me that he knew a man who had the same cancer as I have. He told me that the guy was still living, and that was thirteen years ago. A good-looking young lady pulled me off to the side and told me that she had cancer in the past. Now she was doing fine. She told me, in essence, to keep my head and hope up. "God got you, and I will keep you in my prayers."

The timeline of my treatments was the summer of 2019. I couldn't ride that John Deere zero-turn mower to cut my lawn. Thank God for my great neighbor, a young family man, a truck driver, who told me not to worry, as he would keep my lawn cut. That he did. It was now hot June to July 2019. I was now halfway through what was to be eight treatments of chemotherapy and infusion. I was noticing that my tongue was getting blacker. My fingernails were turning dark.

My hair didn't fall out. I was told that it wouldn't fall out, but it became very silky and soft. During Fourth of July time frame, my sisters from Sacramento, California, and southern Mississippi visited me. I love to cook, so I mustered up enough strength to help prepare a nice meal for them. To see me sick, weak, and not feeling the best was a new experience for them. Then to know I was suffering from pancreatic cancer was a bomber. We ate, and at times I would try to tell them some of what I was going through and experiencing. At the time of their departure, the food in my stomach and the side effects of the chemo caused me to cramp terribly. I wanted to walk out to the car with them for my farewell speech—"Thank y'all for coming, and be safe." I had to turn around and stay inside because I was in such pain and agony of the chemo side effects. I had to cry! Men, don't let your pride get you. Cry. Let it out. Don't be ashamed. Going through the ordeal of pancreatic cancer and chemotherapy will cause one to cry. Going through my treatments and the scans, drinking contrast water, and doing blood work and infusion caused me to reflect and thank God for the experience and all the people sent to wish me well. I even had to pray for me too. I prayed for others also.

These diverse cancers have no respect for people. I sat beside those going through treatments. They were young, old, black, white, male, female, Asian, Latino, East Indian, and so on. I even saw members of my church family whom I didn't know were going through treatments. During my treatments I would carry my Sunday school book and Bible to help me get through the four hours or so of infusion. My eyes were opened. I observed that there was a huge number of blacks doing jobs in the medical profession that I didn't even know existed—infusion nurses, phlebotomists, oncologists, anesthesiologists, and many more. Some of these people were even cancer survivors themselves. These first-line caregivers were compassionately on the job. I loved kidding around with the volunteer workers who were just gladly there in the treatment center, freely giving their time to pass out chips, water, soft drinks, and cookies for the clients' comfort. I probed. They, too, had wonderful stories to tell. Hearing those stories helped me tremendously to take the focus off myself and to look at those who were going through the same ordeal as me.

Some of the patients had seniority, meaning they had been in treatments longer than me, and there were those who started treatments after I did. This kind of ranking gave me great hope that I would finish the treatments also. I saw a young grandson sitting patiently with his grandmother going through her infusion. I heard a man tell the story that he was a gambler and how he had to fight to get home. Whatever place where he gambled, he claimed there was a tough black woman whom no one would dare to mess with. Another elderly man who was going through treatments had a close friend as his caregiver and fishing partner. From her, I learned the directions to their favorite fishing hole. I also sat beside those who said, "If it hadn't been for the Affordable Care Act, I wouldn't have known what to do." During treatments people shared some of their many interesting life stories.

In some ways, the agony of treatments aside, going through my chemotherapy and infusion treatments was interesting, educational, and uplifting. I have learned, as I drove or rode down those double-wide streets and boulevards, to not take for granted when you see clusters of joined together one-story buildings with signs that read Gastro-One, Oncology, Cancer Center, and other specialized medical treatments. Their parking lots are full of cars, but there are very few people outside. The people are there but inside, going through various life-saving efforts to get help dealing with a variety of cancers. Let's open our eyes and understand what's going on inside and offer to help. A case of ginger ale to help with nausea, a twelve-pack small chips, or a few hours of volunteer work that I saw bring great comfort to those going through various cancer treatments.

I had been going through treatments now for several weeks and could see and appreciate the help given. It was now late summer 2019. I had learned the pattern and the ability to deal with it in a positive way. It was now time to check on Alex Trebek's condition and progress. I was diagnosed just two months after him. It was announced that he was stage four; therefore, I always felt that I could see how he was doing to gauge and determine my progress. I googled him. I found my experiences and symptoms were very much in line with his, such as the yellowing of the skin and the eyes. I saw where someone spoke of the terrible experiences of the "bilirubin" agony. Like Alex, I felt the need to be positive and to keep active. In his case it looked like he wanted to keep working. I found that to be very interesting. Based on my observations, those whom I have known to have pancreatic cancer were busy and very active people. In fact, I was told to be active and to stay mobile as long as I possibly could. I will caution us all, though, not to be too active and busy to check out fully the red flags that are common to those of us who have been diagnosed with pancreatic cancer so that we don't let something sneak up on us. So to actors, singers, politicians, musicians, sport broadcasters, and those of us who work several jobs and are approaching age sixty, slow down and smell the roses. Listen to your body. This could mean the difference in detecting something early and stage four. Your mind will surely mess with you. It will tell you, "I told you last year to go and get a checkup."

Through it all, like Trebek, I had hope. I knew that this was a deadly cancer. It fell on me like a ton of bricks out of nowhere. In view of a low survival rate for this cancer, Trebek showed me great courage and strength to want to stay in the fight and continue to work as he was in the fight of his life. I watched him continue to do *Jeopardy!* and the Colonial Penn commercial until it reached $9.95 per unit. That encouraged me tremendously. As long as I could, I continued to play trombone in a local community band. I stayed active in my church work. I even got up enough strength to do a Sunday school lesson at my church. Again, Trebek seemed to talk openly and frankly about his condition and what he was going through. I was observing him closely because I was just two months behind him. I, too, talked openly about my pancreatic cancer. I told the mailman, my church brethren, my neighbors, the pastor, the barber, and even the people at my local cleaners. My wife would check me and ask me, "Why do you tell everybody you have pancreatic cancer?" To talk about it and tell others was a great therapy for me. I had a testimony, and I would hear testimonials from others. Among all those people, I discovered that many of them had been touched or affected by one of the many cancer diseases. These exchanges provided uplift and encouragement to me and them. They also provided me with that great cloud of witnesses and prayers to God for my strength and healing. This also gave me the opportunity to listen and hear about the afflictions of others and the chance to encourage and pray for others even as I was going through my trials of pancreatic cancer. I needed mental, physical, and spiritual strength to endure the task. Talking about it openly was very positive for me.

It was now late summer of 2019. I was nearing the last chemo infusion. In fact, as I was released from the infusion pump of my sixth treatment, I was told by my oncologist's nurse practitioner that I was finished with chemotherapy. I thought she was joking. I was prepared to do number seven. But it was real! I said, "No mo' chemo." That was a great relief and great news to hear. I had completed the first phase of my treatment. I was informed that I would have a few weeks to let my body rebound and strengthen up from the effects of chemotherapy. This marked the beginning of phase two of my treatment sandwich, the radiation with chemo pill part. The interim period between these two phases of my treatment allowed me to reflect on how I was doing and feeling. I looked back on how I sat among other patients going through the same or very similar treatments and situations. They were younger, older, males and females, all creeds and colors, and in various conditions. Seeing this helped me take the focus off myself and to feel compassion for others. This gave me the opportunity to secretly pray to God for his strength to be given to us to help us endure what we were experiencing. During this interim period, I also saw the effects of chemotherapy subside. My tongue, gums, fingernails, and palms began to change from black to their normal color. Also my jaundice eyes were turning to their normal color. The people whom I told that I had completed chemotherapy were telling me that I would be all right. Some were saying, "Don't claim that. You will be around here for a long time." I was told to keep mobile as long as I could. All the positive comments and prayers kept me positive and very hopeful for the best outcome of this fight that I was in.

PHASE TWO: RADIATION THERAPY

It was now time for me to meet with the radiation oncologist, a member of the team assigned to me for my treatment plan. This was all new to me. I was too green to be afraid. A few months earlier, I had been diagnosed with pancreatic cancer. I'd heard of it and cancer in general, yet truthfully, I still didn't know what it was. However, I had the scars and proof of treatments and chemotherapy that let me know it was real. As my pastor often said, "You don't know *it's true* until it happens *to you*." I was encouraged during my first briefing with the radiation oncologist. He stated to me that he was there not just to treat the cancer but also to cure it. Just as I heard people say, "Don't claim that," or, "You'll be around here for a long time," I took the doctor's words as another confirmation that I was and would be okay. It was explained to me that the purpose of the radiation therapy was to shrink further the cancerous tumor so the surgeon would have success in completely getting rid of it. It was further explained to me that radiation therapy would be done five days a week for six weeks. I was also assured that it would not be as rough on me as chemotherapy, though I was given chemo pills to go along with radiation. I was told that this treatment would be pinpointed only to the cancerous tumor. I would have no skin burns or scarring. On subsequent appointments I was marked on my stomach and sides for the accuracy, pinpointing the radiation only to where it was needed. My hat is tipped, and my big thank you goes out to those professional technicians in radiation therapy who did their jobs with grace.

The distance from my home to the radiation center was greater than fifty miles one way. This drive would be a great challenge for me to do because of my weakened state of health. Also my wife's sense of direction is very poor. This drive would have made us both very nervous and uncomfortable driving in the heavy traffic in and around the corridors of Memphis I-55, I-240, and I-40 back and forth twice daily for six weeks. I had been told that lodging and transportation was available to patients who were more than fifty miles away. After my first trip with my car, I told my wife I was signing up for the lodging and transportation benefit. Oh, that became a big part of my treatment experiences. I got billeting in a place called Harrah's Hope Lodge, a place donated by charity. I was able to see and experience the gift of charity and voluntary contributions made to various cancer societies. Harrah's Hope Lodge was located right next to Sun Studio, close to Beale Street and the FedExForum. The drivers who transported me and others to the various treatment sites were volunteers. Many of them were cancer survivors themselves. I know that they don't realize how much comfort they give. I learned a lot from talking to them and seeing the value of their freely given time to bring hope to us.

I got the chance to visit the Sun Studio and hold and sing in the mike that was donated and held by Elvis Presley. One volunteer driver was a member of a small group that regularly gathered together in a small pub close to the FedExForum to eat catfish, chicken wings, and fries and discuss the outcome of a current FedExForum event. This small pub was recommended to my wife and me as a place to visit and to eat while going through my treatments. We tried it, and we were not disappointed. I also had the chance to walk a little on Beale Street, where I saw this one man who had a great voice singing the blues. I started to hum along with him. That was fun and a great joy for me. He asked my wife and me where we lived. I told him, and that allowed me the opportunity to let even the blues man know that I was a man experiencing and going through pancreatic cancer and treatments. That blessed us both—I received his well-wishes, and he got mine.

The actual radiation therapy process wasn't bad at all. It was daily, though short. Again, I sat beside men and women, young and old, going through the same radiation therapy as me for the same or similar cancers. I had been marked for pinpointed accuracy. I would watch how the radiation technicians would align those light beams and adjust my body for the accuracy of the radiation to hit only those places where it was directed. Again, I got no burn or scarring on my body externally. As the radiation equipment was set and I was accurately aligned, my mental prayer would be for the technicians. I thanked God for giving them the knowledge, skill, desire, and wisdom to do such a great work as his extenders to care for and treat his people. I heard the sounds and changes in the sounds of the radiation machine as it rotated around my body from left to right. I would meditate deeply, daily, during my radiation therapy. I would say, "Lord, guide those radiation beams directly to where they need to go for me as well as for others. In my case kill this cancer and throw it in the Coldwater River to raise its head no more." Every now and then, I had to remind myself that I was a pancreatic cancer patient even when I tried to find joy in this ordeal I was experiencing.

I was now approaching the end of my radiation therapy. It was a great experience. All the radiation technicians were young, energetic, polite, and professional. I thank God for all of them for their great work. I appreciate very much the great conversations I had with other patients about their experiences as we waited for our time to be called in for treatment. You have become my mental friends. I don't know your names or where you are from, but I do remember mentally your faces. I still pray for you and wonder where you are and how you are doing. The many volunteers, the churches, the university students, many of whom are studying to care for cancer patients. I even became a friend of Ensure vanilla and chocolate drinks. You allowed me to see Shelby Farms Park. I thank you all, and I thank God so very much for you all.

My last week of radiation was upon me. There was this one radiation technician who would pump me up and cheer me on, telling me, "Hey, Friday is your last day. You see that big bell? You will get to ring it!" I had heard the sound of that bell ringing before by those who rang it before me. I did get to that Friday, my last day of radiation therapy. I told others that it was my last day of treatments. This was to encourage others who had started treatments after me to hang in there, as I was encouraged by those who started and finished ahead of me. Wow! I rang that big bell! What a great milestone I had reached in my treatment plan. I had already completed a series of chemo treatments. Now I was ringing the bell, indicating that I had successfully completed the radiation therapy phase, a big part of my treatment plan. This was a celebration. The hand-claps and congratulatory greetings from the radiation technicians, my wife, and those who sat beside me awaiting their time were all a great source

MY TREATMENT PLAN

of strength and hope to me. I thank you all so very much. You have become my mental friends.

I was now back under the control of the oncologist. I met again with this doctor to get further explanation of my treatment plan. First thing, as always, I got blood work and a CAT scan done to determine how I was doing internally. My blood work was declared to be good, and all my numbers were in balance. My blood pressure was good, glucose was a little high, red and white blood cells were good, and overall I felt fairly good, though still a little weak. I did those things that I thought would keep me going. I went fishing, I looked for garage sales, and I read my Bible. I also made calls to friends and relatives and watched the news. My oncologist further explained to me that my treatment would continue to be like building a sandwich. I had chemotherapy, the foundation or the bottom slice. On it, the radiation therapy with oral chemo pills were placed. I had just completed that phase. Now the oncologist explained that surgery would be the meat part of the sandwich or the third phase of my treatment plan, where the cancerous tumor would be surgically removed. The oncologist set up an appointment for me to meet again with the surgeon. However, I was given an interim period before the appointment. This period was given to allow my body to heal even more, gain strength, and recuperate further from the rough period of chemotherapy and radiation therapy.

During this period I did feel my energy level get better. I saw my hands, fingernails, tongue, eyes, and gums go back to their normal color. You know the saying, "I looked at my hands, and they looked new. I looked at my eyes, and they did too"? It was now around September to October 2019. I was diagnosed just two months after Alex Trebek's diagnosis. Unknowingly to him, he became my mental friend. During this interim period, I felt that it was time to google Alex Trebek to see how he was doing. I felt that the way he was doing would be a way to measure how I was doing. I found out I also had the same or similar pain and agony he wrestled with. I was encouraged by his boldness to openly talk about his struggle with this dreadful pancreatic cancer. I was also glad to share with anyone the experiences of my battle. I hope that I am a mental mentor to someone who is suffering this mean disease. Please pray for and be a mental friend to someone who is not aware of your friendship. Being an adult, I am now realizing that our children who are struggling with diverse cancers need our prayers and support to help them battle these terrible diseases also.

The time had arrived that I consulted with my surgeon again. It was decision time—do surgery or do not do surgery. The timeline was very close to Christmas. I had been waiting and waiting and praying to God for a clear mind to make a clear decision about my next step. At such a time, I had to be still and think for myself. There were those who would tell me, "Man, I wouldn't do that." Others would say, "They just want to cut on you because they think you have pretty good insurance." No, I have pancreatic cancer! I want this demon off me. I had to put negative clutter out of my mind and rely on my faith in God to give me the right mind to make the right decision.

PHASE THREE: THE SURGICAL PHASE

I NOW FOUND MYSELF MEETING AND speaking again with the surgeon, the same surgeon I had spoken with earlier and gained confidence in him. He had a diagram of what looked like the whole digestive system, with the liver, intestines, gallbladder, and pancreas. These were inner parts I knew I had but hadn't given much thought to their significance. I supposed I had taken the importance of these inner parts for granted. The surgeon showed me that he would surgically remove the tumor, clip the head of the pancreas, remove the gallbladder, and do a few other things with my intestines. Then he would put me back together again. In layman's terms that was how I understood what was explained to me. The surgeon was concerned that the tumor was very close to some vital blood vessels. That made me realize how important both the chemotherapy and radiation therapy were in shrinking the tumor so the surgeon would have working room.

My oncologist had already explained to me that I was facing a very serious operation. This operation was the same as or greater than open-heart surgery. The oncologist further explained that if she had to have the exact procedure done on her, she would have the same surgeon I had to perform it. The surgery prescribed for me was the "Whipple procedure." It was now decision time to have this procedure done. It was now late 2019, approaching Christmas. I had some time to think about it. However, I felt my decision had already been made. I had prayed to God for a clear mind to make a clear decision according to his will. I didn't have a struggle with the little man in my head where I would think *yes* and the little man would say *no* or vice versa. When people would ask how I was doing, I would explain to them what I was faced with and say that I was going to have surgery sometime around the Christmas holidays.

Even when I discussed the situation with my wife, I would say, "Honey, my mind is made up. I am going to have the surgery."

Then she would say, "Well, I don't want this to linger and be carried over into the new year." We agreed to spend Christmas together at home.

I called the surgeon and asked for the first available surgery date between Christmas and the new year. The surgeon mustered up his team and told my wife and me to be prepared and ready to go at approximately 5:30 a.m. on December 31, 2019, New Year's Eve. Later, I realized what great timing it was. After a forty-five-minute drive, I arrived at the hospital. It was cold, and I felt a little weak. However, I was in good spirits and unafraid. My mind was completely clear of negative thoughts and useless clutter. It was like being seated on an airplane and you see the flight attendant close the door shut. Then you realize your fate is with God, the pilots, and the aircraft. I was now at the hospital and placed in my little cubicle on a stretcher. I was asked to state my name and date of birth for verification.

I was now fully into phase three of my treatment plan, the surgery phase. Two from my church family arrived to be with my wife and me to cheer us on and to offer encouragement and well-wishes at five a.m., on cold New Year's Eve! I am forever grateful to them for their love and kindness. I was laughing and talking with them while at the same time talking with the medical personnel and anesthesiologists. I was very pleased and happy to see again the number of blacks in high-ranking positions in the medical field, such as registered nurses, anesthesiologists, and operating room specialists.

My intake process went smoothly and fairly quickly. The well-wishes, kisses, and holding of my hands had come to a close. I saw and felt myself being rolled down the corridors of the hospital and into a well-lighted room. I was surrounded by several operating room specialists. I was pulled off the stretcher and placed onto an operating table. I remember well how painstakingly I was placed on that table. While on my back, I gazed up at those huge round lights while at the same time observing how well those medical workers were performing their jobs, working well together. I was smiling and somewhat laughing to myself. I had to have a good sense of humor. I was asking myself, "Boy, what in the world have you gotten yourself into?" I realized that this was it. I was being made ready to be cut on. Like when the doors of the airplane are shut and you are on it, I knew then that I was in the hand of God and his extenders, the medical personnel who were assigned to me for my care. I had prayed for that. I heard, "Turn your head and breathe right here normally." It seemed like I was breathing in a soft mist. I was smiling and saying to myself, "This stuff ain't gonna put me to sleep." That was the last thing I remembered. Then the long blank.

Some five-and-a-half hours later, I found myself back where I started from, back on the stretcher in my recovery cubicle. I began to wake up. I saw people but faintly. I heard my name being called. I was asked questions to see if I was awake and alert. I was gaining consciousness and becoming well aware of my surroundings. I noticed the time on the clock was a long ways away from five a.m. I don't recall the first time I saw my wife at that point of my recovery. The next thing I realized was that I was all tubed up and in ICU on New Year's Day. So happy New Year 2020! My ICU experience was pleasant. I felt I was in a first-class seat of the hospital. A few days later, I found myself in a regular room in a regular bed. First class was over.

Now I remember very well when my wife showed up. She decorated my room with nice little things to look at. She brought all kinds of sweet scents that had my room smelling good. Nurses and hospital custodians would come in and comment on how good my room looked and smelled. Still tubed and stapled up, it seemed the emphasis was, "Hurry up and get better so you can go home." "Get him up" and "Sit him up" seemed to be the orders of the day. Daily, I felt better than the day before. Shortly, the tube through my nose and into my throat was taken out. Boy, I was glad to get rid of that. The drainage tubes in my left and right side, one after the other, were taken out. Then the stitches and staples were dealt with. "Get up, sit up. Your doctor doesn't want to come in and find you in bed, okay?" I was good with that. So I had to walk.

Other than the physical therapist, there was this one person who saw to it that I had towels and clean linens. She told me that I was doing so well that she would walk with me daily. She did, and I walked even farther than was expected. She told me I was doing extremely well and progressing greatly for the type of surgery I had, and for my age. She told me to hurry up so I could go home. She expressed to me that I would do so much better in my home environment. My doctor, the surgeon, told me that I was doing well. He told me that if I kept it up, he might let me have a Popsicle tomorrow.

I now started to hear rumors of a discharge date. After several days in the hospital, though not that long, I was de-tubed, sat up, walked up and down the corridors of my hospital floor, and handed towels and bodywash to bathe myself with. In other words I had recuperated enough. It was time for me to go home. I was told several times that patients did better at home than in the hospital environment. This was late January 2020 time frame. The noise of the coronavirus was getting louder and louder. I discerned that the medical people knew more about it than me. The emphasis at this time seemed to have been mainly on hand-washing, gloves, and sanitizer.

The big day finally arrived, the day I was to have conference with the surgeon to talk about being discharged from the hospital. It was on the same day that my wife and church friend visited me. They had been with me for a couple of hours. When they were preparing to leave for home, I told them to hold up and wait with me a little while longer. I assured them that the doctor would be in at any moment. I wanted my wife to be with me and to hear what the doctor would say about how I was doing and when I would possibly be going home.

Finally, the doctor arrived. He spoke and greeted my wife and friend. After a word with them, he turned and placed his attention on me. He asked how I was doing. I replied that I was doing okay and ready to eat a meal. He sat down beside me and stated that the chemo and radiation therapy had worked in shrinking my tumor. He told us that the tumor had shrunk down to about the size of a pea. He asked if I had a piece of paper. All I had was my Sunday school book, so I turned it to a page that had been left blank on purpose. He began to demonstrate and sketch a small pea-size circle. He stated the tumor had shrunk down to seven millimeters. This shrinkage gave him room to work around those delicate blood vessels he had told me about before surgery. He also told us that he checked not one, not five, but eleven lymph nodes and found none to be cancerous.

Wow! I didn't understand all that. I just asked, "Doc, did you get it all?"

His reply was "All I saw."

"Doc, how about my gallbladder?"

He told me that he got all that out too and dropped it into the bucket. That was when the tears of joy started to roll down my face. We all started to thank God and to give him the glory for all he had done, is doing, and going to do as I further my journey to get my life back. The doctor told me that I was doing well and would be going home tomorrow.

Five minutes later, my pastor surprisingly walked in to visit me. I was located on the fifth floor of the hospital.

I said, "Pastor, if you had been here five minutes earlier and heard what the doctor had told us, you would have jumped out of that window for joy. The doctor told me that he had got that cancer out of me!"

Wow! There went another loud shout of praise to the Lord with even more prayer and tears of joy.

The chemo and radiation therapy had done their job. The cancerous tumor was diminished down to seven millimeters, which allowed the surgeon ample room to work around those delicate blood vessels without disturbing them. The surgeon told me that he checked several lymph nodes and found none to be cancerous.

The next day finally arrived. It was time to gladly go home to further recuperate. I said my thanks and goodbyes to the on-duty staff. I was wheelchaired out of the hospital to my awaiting car. I was discharged with only three very small pain pills and a handheld respirator. There was no chance of me getting hooked on pills. At home now! I was very sore and weak. I had to learn how to get in and out of bed again. That was where my patient caregiving wife was a big help and a great blessing. I was also assigned with a home health nurse and a physical therapist. These two were very helpful also. The nurse would check my vital signs and kept a close eye on me. The physical therapist was great also. When I was ready, he gradually introduced me to various exercises to build my strength up so I could better become independent to get in and out of bed, go to the bathroom, and walk. I was down to about 220 pounds from 270 before my diagnosis. What a terrible weight-loss program; however, I did lose weight.

The timeline now was around the latter part of February and into the first of March 2020. The noise of the coronavirus was getting even louder as well as the American politics, the 2020 presidential election. I alluded to this earlier that my timing was great. I was in and out of the hospital for the most part when the real weight of the COVID-19 hit. That provided me a ringside seat in front of the fireplace with the TV remote in hand, flipping back and forth from local news to the breaking news of CNN. In other words I was "glued to the tube" as I was recuperating from my pancreatic cancer surgery.

Also I had heard bits and pieces about the coronavirus while in the hospital. However, at that time no one was wearing masks. Though I did notice the wearing of gloves and the washing of hands with the use of hand sanitizer being practiced more. Looking back, I think that the hospital knew something was brewing as it related to the coronavirus that I, the patient, didn't know. The guidance and guidelines on how to deal with the virus were not clear or well defined then. I put a mask on one day. I was asked by my nurse on duty why I was wearing that mask. I didn't answer clearly because I didn't want to offend anyone. The reason I wore the mask was that I smelled what I thought was a sniff of a bad sinus infection. I didn't want to catch a cold and get pneumonia where I would have had to do a lot of coughing that would have been very painful with a new surgery. Therefore, I wore that mask and puffed on that little respirator given to me to keep my chest and lungs open.

At the time I didn't know that later I would be classified as a person with underlying conditions. I was slowly weaned from my home health nurse and physical therapist, and to both I owe a great deal of gratitude for their great assistance in being the first line in my postoperative at-home recovery. I saw them stressing the use of gloves and bringing in small tubes of hand sanitizer because of the fact that this coronavirus was going to be very serious. I was glued to the tube as I was getting stronger daily. I was hearing and seeing on TV how fast this virus was spreading. I heard many rumors of where it might have started. I saw many people contracting it and dying from it. Naturally I was very concerned because of the fact that I had just had pancreatic cancer surgery and was afraid of getting pneumonia.

My glucose level was running a bit high, so I requested an appointment with my primary care doctor to get an A1C test. On the day of my exam, I noticed that I had to remain in my car. I was greeted through my car window by my physician, dressed in full personal protective equipment or PPE, a term I learned from watching the TV. I was asked what I was doing there. I replied that I had an appointment for an A1C test. After a quick stick on the finger, I was told that I was okay and to go home and that I didn't need to be out there. That was when I realized the weight of COVID-19 was real.

The timeline now was somewhere around the latter part of April and early May 2020. I had begun to be more mobile and to do some of those things I had done before on a limited and how-I-felt basis. Using my cane, I would walk to soak up the early spring sun. I would drive short distances. I even went back to my church. I think I even mustered up enough strength to teach a Sunday school class and thank God and the brethren for their prayers and support. Stronger in strength spiritually, mentally, and physically, it was now time that my oncologist called me in for checkup and counsel.

PHASE FOUR: CONTINUING MY TREATMENT PLAN

I SAT DOWN WITH MY ONCOLOGIST. She again unfolded the strategy of my treatment plan, which she likened to building a sandwich.

MY TREATMENT PLAN

She explained that the first slice was the chemotherapy and infusion treatments. On top of that, I had a phase of successive pinpointed radiation therapy with chemo pills treatments. The meat of the treatment plan was the surgery. I successively completed those phases. Now to cap the treatment plan off, I was told that I had six more chemotherapy with infusion treatments to go. Wow! That was a bitter pill to swallow. Like a man, with God's help and strength, I was able to do it.

COVID-19 was now loud and wreaking havoc in America and around the world. During this round of chemo treatments, I left my wife at home because of the dangers of COVID-19. One had to be masked up, checked for temperature, and socially distanced. In addition the politics of America was very loud and heated as I was counting down my treatments. There was this elderly lady who had been in her series of last chemo treatments longer than me. Therefore, she completed her treatments ahead of me. When she had finished her last treatment, the infusion nurse made the announcement to all that the lady had completed her last treatment. She then was permitted to write her name on a wall of names of those who had done it before. The infusion nurse declared her to be a cancer survivor. She was then allowed to ring the huge bell. What great joy to behold! I too had hope. The wells of my eyes just overflowed with tears joy for her. The infusion nurse comforted me and told me that *I would ring that bell too*. In September 2020 I was declared a pancreatic cancer survivor! I too *rang that bell*. That was the top slice of my treatment sandwich. Lord, I thank you. I give you all the glory.

REFLECTIONS

I LOOK AT MY PANCREATIC CANCER experience and count it as part of my life. I am humbled by the fact that I still have a port in my chest and a long surgical scar on my stomach that will be with me for the rest of my life. I still hear the sound of my surgeon in my head saying I could die from it and that it could come back. I also heard him say after a year I would be getting my life back. I also saw and heard in God's Word that he is an ever-present help in times of trouble, a deliverer and healer. What an experience! Looking back, that was a hard row to hoe. Without God's help and strength, I couldn't have made it alone. With joy, I can now laugh about it. I tell myself the roughest parts about it were the agony of constipation, the bilirubin that caused me to itch and feel as if little demons were trying to escape through my skin, and the chemotherapy. The lightest parts were the radiation therapy and the surgery. During radiation I had access to and the benefits of Harrah's Hope Lodge. The lodge provided lodging and transportation to and from radiation treatments. The great volunteer drivers, some of whom were survivors themselves, drove us through the scenic routes of Memphis and Shelby Farms. During surgery I was asleep and felt no pain.

When I was going through my ordeal, I became a mental prayer warrior, silently interceding on behalf of those who sat beside me in treatment going through the same or similar situation as me. Alex Trebek, I will remember him. He was diagnosed with pancreatic cancer in March 2019, just two months before me. I tried to keep a close eye on him and watch his progress and hear what he was experiencing and doing that would help me get through my fight. Then I saw where President Obama had invited Aretha Franklin to perform at the Kennedy Center Honors. I believe I noticed some of the physical scars this dreaded pancreatic cancer had on her, yet her voice was still strong, and she was engaged in her gift. During her performance I seemed to have heard her say something like no matter what the doctors might say, God had the last word. Oh, what great strength and comfort that gave to me. That sentiment was incorporated into my way of thinking that kept me positive.

In August 2018 the Alpha and Omega spoke. Then I observed the great and strong Ruth Bader Ginsburg struggling with her diseases. I saw how she kept working until the end. On December 30, 2019, just one day before my pancreatic surgery, I learned that Representative John Lewis had announced that he had stage four pancreatic cancer. Deeper on into the year 2020, still glued to the tube, I saw and heard how Representative Lewis proclaimed his many fights while at the same time realizing that pancreatic cancer was a different kind of demon to wrestle with. I liked his spirit. He kept on dancing and doing his work. "Get into good trouble," he said. I say when one gets into good trouble, keep dancing, keep working, and keep hoping they will get out of good trouble. He got out in July 2020.

My main measuring stick was Alex Trebek. He left us in November 2020, just two months after I was declared a pancreatic cancer survivor. Unknowingly to him, he was my mental partner and encourager, and I was his mental prayer warrior. I have learned that Count Basie, the famous musician; Patrick Swayze and Brock Peters, both actors; and Pavarotti, a great singer, fought this terrible disease. Now, those mentioned were widely known individuals. Now that I am in the midst, I can list those who are not so widely known, such as the Leroys, the Eds, the dads, the Felicias, Cousin Edna's mom, the many who didn't even know they had this demonic pancreatic cancer, and me.

The timeline now is around late September 2020 through January 2021. COVID-19 is now a pandemic that is wreaking havoc in America and around the world. Because of the 2020 presidential election race, American politics is very loud and something to behold. Mask wearing, glove wearing, temperature checking, social distancing, and the politics of the day are all playing a part in my getting my life back.

THE WONDERMENT

THIS PANCREATIC CANCER DISEASE CAME upon me like a ton of bricks out of nowhere. The question I asked was why I didn't know it before now. The answer was there are no symptoms, and any time after age sixty, one can expect anything to happen to them. I won't argue the point with the experts; however, as the one who contracted the disease, I wonder whether I had symptoms or saw or felt any signs of the disease on me before diagnosis. Personally I feel that I saw plenty of signs and symptoms. I just didn't know what they were or how to process them. I had weight gain, weakness in my left thigh, red eyes, dark and heavy-looking urine, and uncontrollable gas. I also had anxiety spells and periods of heavy daytime tiredness or sleepiness. I wondered many times why I got sleepy while waiting for a traffic light to change. Can you imagine yourself going to sleep while riding on a John Deere zero-turn lawn mower and waking up going around and around in circles?

I went to the doctors for these symptoms, even the dark urine. When I went to the doctor to see about my back and weakness in my thigh, blood work was done. It was the vigilance of that doctor who reviewed the results of my blood work and saw that my liver enzymes were very high, then personally called me to tell me to go straight to the emergency room. I wonder where I would be today if that had not happened. I also wonder if doctors and medical personnel would be more vigilant in looking at patients' test results, would they find conditions earlier? I was asked several times if anyone in my family had pancreatic cancer. Quickly I would say no because I didn't know. In my case I remembered hearing my sister say my dad had a spot somewhere in his stomach. The doctors would give him blood. It quickly passed through him. Those facts made me wonder what my dad's condition was. Therefore, I ordered his death certificate to satisfy my curiosity. Guess what. The cause of death was pancreatic cancer. In addition to getting obituaries, I now say to family members get the death certificates of your loved ones. Evaluate and know the cause of death. This possibly could help the doctors better look for markers to better treat you.

I read in scripture that we are made with knowledge, skill, and wisdom. It even declares that we are wonderfully made. I often wonder if the problems that I was having, that I considered as possible signs of this cancer, were telling me something was wrong. After I was diagnosed, I went back to one of my doctors for further evaluation. I told him since I had been diagnosed with pancreatic cancer, the weakness in my left leg that caused me to buckle had stopped. He couldn't explain it, yet he did say our bodies are unique in that one area can indicate a problem elsewhere. Listen to your body, and talk to yourself about what you feel or see. If your head hurts, check it out. Your body could be trying to communicate with you that your blood pressure is up. Report it to your primary care doctor. I wonder if that could mean the difference between no stage and stage four of any disease.

The situations and ordeal I have gone through on the journey to getting my life back cause me to think deeply. I wonder how I'm really doing and progressing. I think of others whom I sat beside during my various treatments. Some had multiple diseases such as diverse cancers along with heart trouble, lung disease, diabetes, and kidney problems. I often wonder how they are doing. There are those who had beat one kind of disease to find themselves faced with a new disease to fight. That is a very humbling experience. Would I have rather had diabetes or kidney cancer? Better yet, would I have done better with prostate cancer or lung cancer? Oh, open-heart surgery might not have been that bad since treatment for that has been greatly advanced. No, being next to it and seeing some of that firsthand, even though rough, I accept the pancreatic cancer and the way God has brought me through it. Did I get a benefit out of my fight with this demonic pancreatic cancer disease? I like to think so. I lost fifty pounds. My glucose runs a bit high; however, my A1C level is good. My blood pressure hangs in good. I keep a check on it, and there is no blood pressure medication. Basically my medication list consists of an antacid pill and a weekly vitamin D pill. Mentally, spiritually, and physically, I feel great.

The noise of COVID-19 has begun to sound softer; however, its presence is still there. Our political climate seems to have gotten better, though there is a dead snake out there that's still wiggling.

I'm getting my life back! I've had days and months of feel-better. I've gone from every three months checkup to every six months now.

On the front end, that sounds very good; however, on the back end, that was kind of scary. I wondered what would go on during those extra three months. It's all good! I've celebrated a couple more birthdays and anniversaries. I am still a mental prayer warrior praying for those who don't even know I'm praying for them. I'm a mentor and encourager to one who heard about me and is now going through the same trial of pancreatic cancer. I am cooking, eating, and going about my business in a positive manner. I even have a pair of tickets to see Smokey Robinson with my wife! Do I have my life back? I give all the glory to God, who is greater than pancreatic cancer.

ACKNOWLEDGMENT

I THANK GOD, HIS BELOVED SON Jesus the Christ, and the Holy Spirit for giving me the power and strength to come into and through this demonic pancreatic cancer trial and tribulation. I thank Jesus Christ for the intimate relationship whereby I felt no shame to pray out to him when I was in trouble. I thank the Holy Spirit that dwells in me, who gave me the right way and eye to look at my situation differently and with the right attitude.

I THANK MY WIFE, MARY BYRD, for being the best caregiver. She put up with the stress of seeing me go through the agony and ordeal of pancreatic cancer.

I THANK SO MUCH ROY POWELL and his mom Linda Powell for driving greater than fifty miles just to support and be with me and my wife New Year's Eve 2019 as I was prepared for surgery. They stayed with me until I was rolled into the operating room. Ain't that "I care about you and love." Sorry to say, in 2020 Roy Powell died of COVID-19.

I THANK RONEY STRONG, SR., MY pastor who prayed and visited me in the hospital.

I AM GRATEFUL TO DR. SUSHMA Chowdhary, my primary care doctor, who diligently reviewed my medical test results, then personally called me and told me to go straight to the emergency room.

I THANK DOCTOR STEPHAN BEHRMAN, MY surgeon, for putting together a great medical team that successfully performed the Whipple procedure on me.

I THANK DR. SONIA BENN, MY oncologist who directed my chemotherapy.

www.ingramcontent.com/pod-product-compliance
Lightning Source LLC
LaVergne TN
LVHW012035060526
838201LV00061B/4623